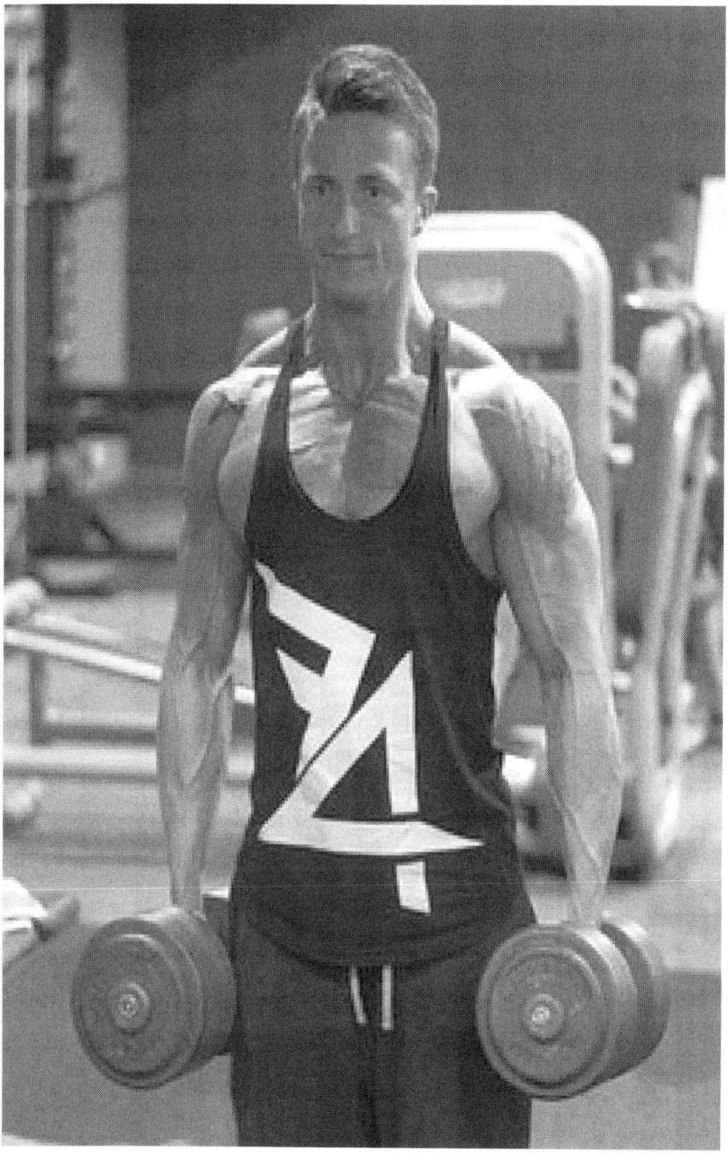

25 BEST DUMBBELL EXERCISES

Dumbbell Exercises for body fitness, Boost Muscles, strength training and Body structure.

STEVE BRIGHT

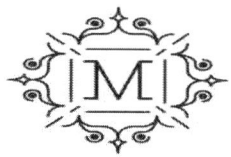

Copyright 2021 Morgan.

This book is subject to copyright policy. All rights are reserved, whether the entire or component of the material, particularly the right of transformation, reprinting, recycling illustration, broadcasting, duplicating on microfilm, or in any other way. No part or even the whole of this book or contents may be produced or even transmitted or reproduced in any way, be it electronic or paper form or by any means, electronic or mechanical, also include recording or by any information storage or retrieval system, without prior written permission the copyright owner, *Morgan LTD.*

TABLE OF CONTENTS

INTRODUCTION 6
PART 1: BASIC UNDERSTANDING DUMBBELL 8
WHAT IS DUMBBELL? 8
BRIEF HISTORY OF DUMBBELL: 10
PART 2: BEST TYPES OF DUMBBELLS. 13
MAIN TYPES OF DUMBBELLS: 14
ADJUSTABLE DUMBBELL: 14
FIXED DUMBBELL: 16
STUDIO DUMBBELL: 17
PART 3: HEALTH BENEFITS OF USING DUMBBELLS
.... 19
PART 4: HOW TO USE DUMBBELL FOR YOUR EXERCISES 22
PART 5: BEST DUMBBELL EXERCISES 24
DUMBBELL BENCH PRESS: 25

GOBLET SQUAT: 26
DUMBBELL CLEAN: 27
DUMBBELL BICEP CURL:..28
SHOULDER PRESS WITH DUMBBELL: 29
BEND OVER ROW:...30
TWO-ARM DUMBBELL STIFF LEGGED DEADLIFT: .31
ONE-ARM SWING: 32
CROSSBODY SINGLE HAMMER CURL:....................33
STEP-UPS WITH DUMBBELL: 34
DUMBBELL SCAPTION:..35
DUMBBELL LUNGE:..36
SINGLE DUMBBELL SHOULDER RAISE: 37
DUMBBELL CALF RAISES:...38
HOLLOW BODY SKULLCRUSHER:............................39
TRICEP KICKBACK: 40
RUSSIAN TWIST: 41
WEIGHT SIT UP/JACK KNIVE:..................................42
LATERAL RAISE DUMBBELL: 43
LYING DUMBBELL FLY:..44
PRESS-UP WITH DUMBBELL:...................................45

INTRODUCTION

Dumbbells are among the most often used items of weight-lifting equipment. Two equivalent weights are mounted to a handle on a dumbbell, as well as the weights may be set or detached. Dumbbells are primarily utilized to strengthen and tone muscles, and they can be used to grow muscles in almost every area of the body. Dumbbells are made up of heavy metal, concrete, and perhaps other materials which come in a variety of weights including sizes.

In this book, we will discuss various exercises you can use a dumbbell to do and also the effect on our body fitness and strength training.

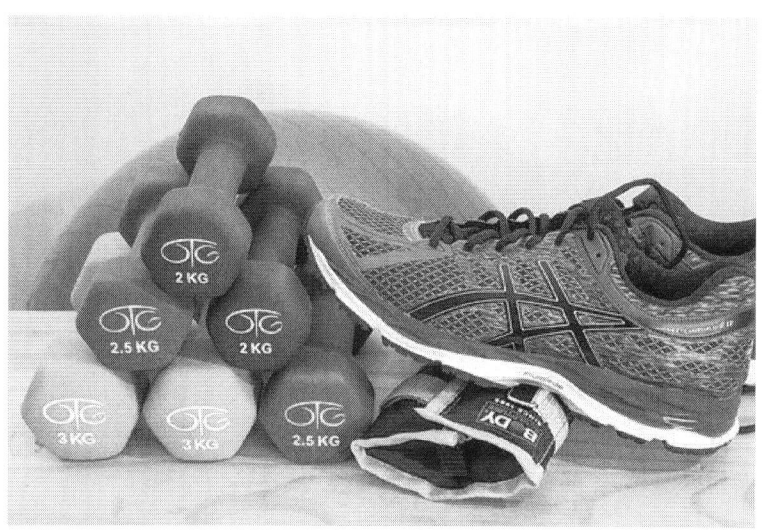

Dumbbells are a good choice for at-home exercises. They are lightweight, cheap, and can be used for a variety of activities that individuals can do in their own homes.

PART 1: BASIC UNDERSTANDING DUMBBELL

In this part, we will discuss the history and basic understanding of what dumbbells can do to our body fitness.

WHAT IS DUMBBELL?

The dumbbell is also known as a free weight. It is a collective piece of equipment mostly used for weight training. Sometimes they are mostly used individually or in sets with one in each of the hands.

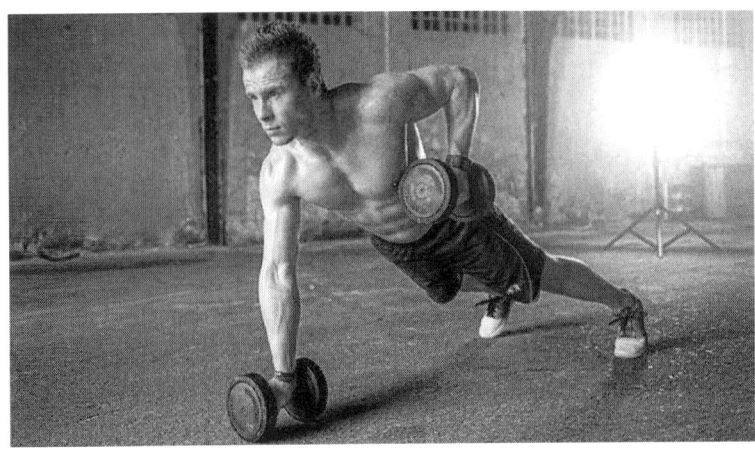

Dumbbells are primarily used for strength training and weight lifting as well as tone muscle.

However, they can be utilized to grow muscles in almost every area of the body. Dumbbells are made up of metal, concrete, including other materials, and they come in a variety of weights including sizes.

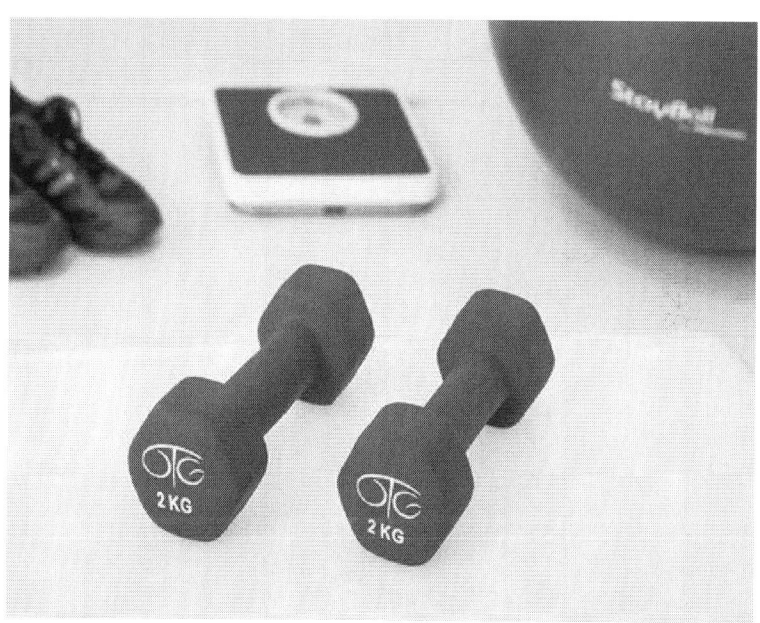

BRIEF HISTORY OF DUMBBELL:

Approximately two thousand years ago, the dumbbell was first brought for the first time. The haltere, a crescent-shaped stone with such a handle developed by the ancient Greeks, was a piece of equipment. This precursor to the dumbbell was utilized as lifting weight and in long jump sports. The "nal" was a further sort of "dumbbell" that was created in prehistoric times.

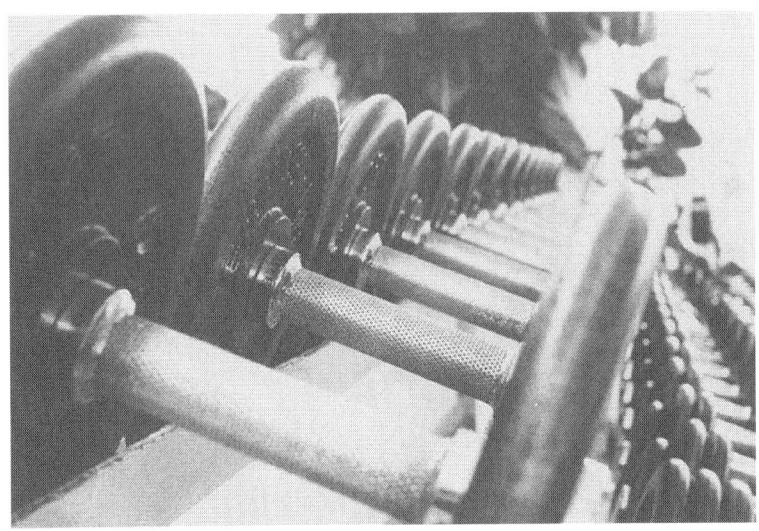

The Indians have been using this equipment for over centuries, and it seemed like a club. Bodybuilders, athletes, and sportsmen used this to develop muscle bulk and stamina since it was wider than a dumbbell but smaller than a barbell.

During the Tudor period in England, the term "dumbbell" was introduced. Athletes used hand-held church bells to strengthen their limbs as well as upper bodies at the time. They wanted to cut the clappers because the bells were causing so much noise during rehearsal. As a result, the bells were "dumb," and the apparatus was dubbed the "dumbbell."

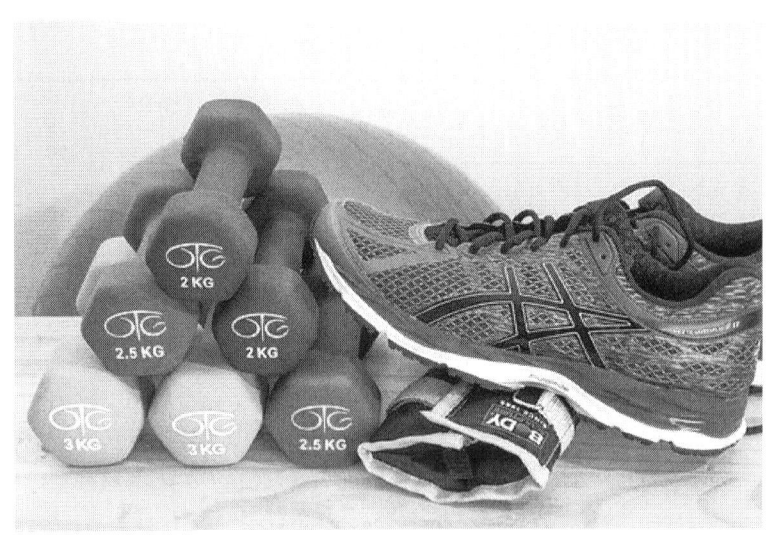

PART 2: BEST TYPES OF DUMBBELLS.

They come in a range of sizes, forms, weights, and materials to meet the needs of different people. They can assist people in saving money on gym memberships while also assisting them in achieving fitness goals like weight loss or muscle growth.

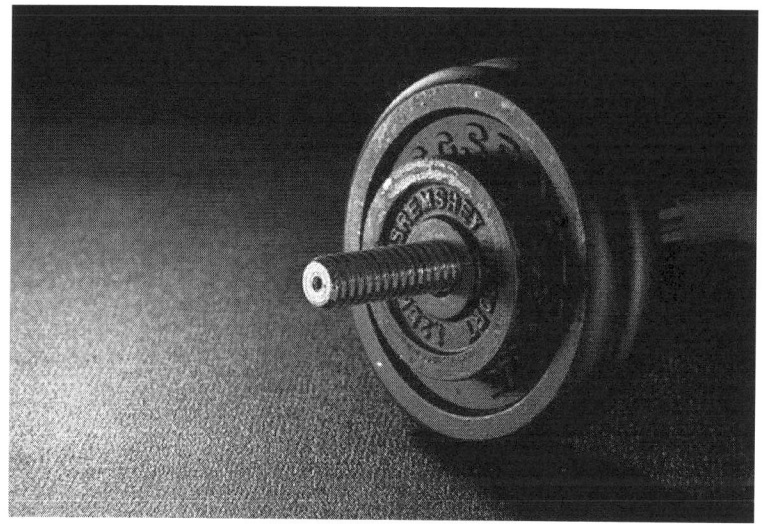

The followings are things you need to consider when buying dumbbell equipment.

- Prices

- Weight and size.
- Your goal and fitness.
- Storage.

MAIN TYPES OF DUMBBELLS:

The followings are the main types of dumbbells:

ADJUSTABLE DUMBBELL:

Dumbbells with adjustable weights allow you to vary or change the volume of weight you're lifting. Bar, as well as plates and classic adjustable dumbbells, are the two main styles of adjustable dumbbells.

Different bars and weight plates enable an individual to increase or decrease weight by adjusting the weight plates.

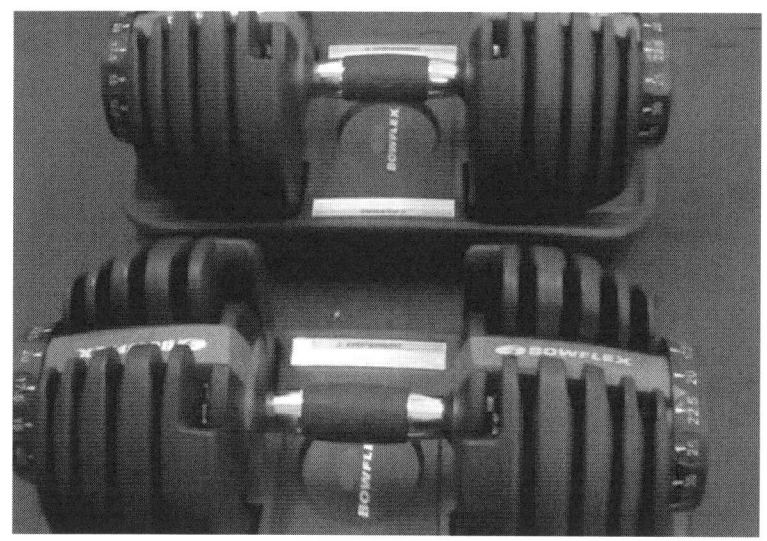

After having to physically add or detach weight plates, the new adjustable style enables individuals to change the weight by pressing and locking well almost weight onto the bar.

These are good options for those who don't have a lot of storage space but want to workout with a range of different weights.

FIXED DUMBBELL:

Dumbbells with a fixed weight have a stable weight. They may be purchased separately, in pairs, or as part of a larger collection. Fixed weights are used in a wide range of products and forms.

Set weights, as opposed to adjustable weights, take up a lot of space to store. As a result, anyone with limited space may want to seek a different alternative.

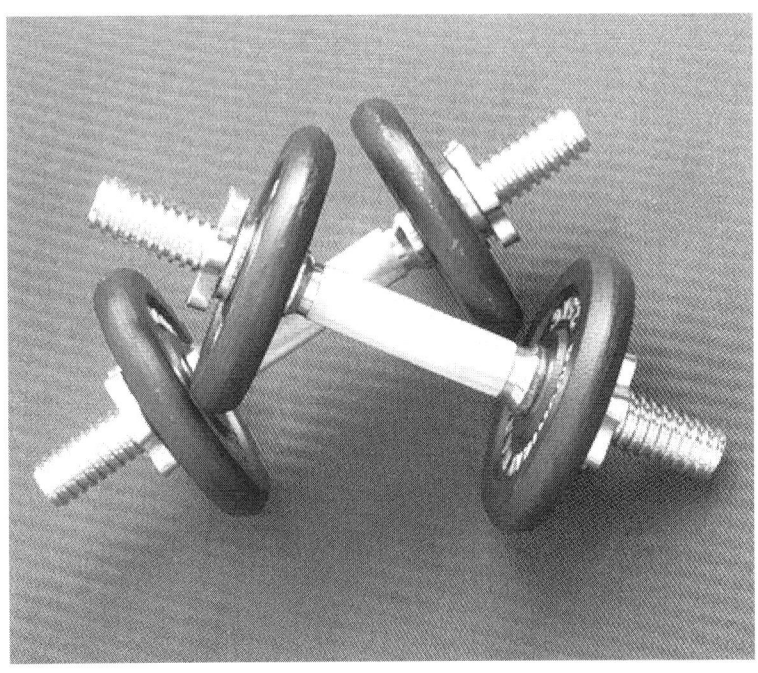

STUDIO DUMBBELL:

Studio weights are usually lighter weights with a textured neoprene or rubber covering. This coating covers the weight while still adding traction.

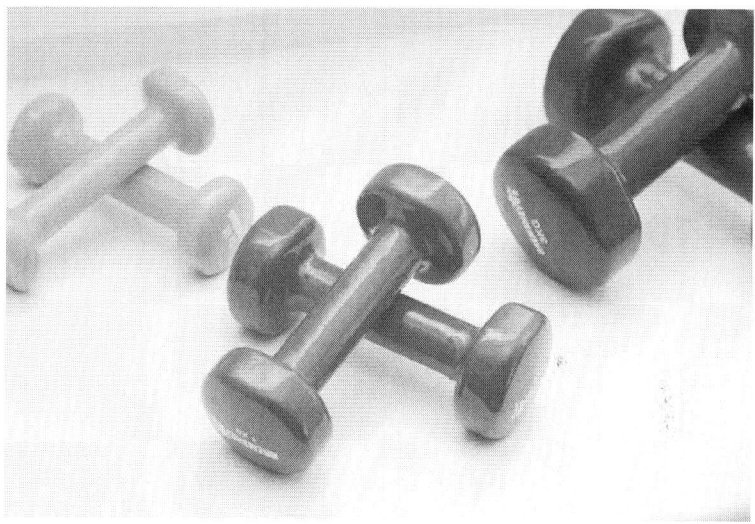

While these weights can be used for strength training, they are a better fit for aerobic workouts due to their lighter weight range and superior grip. Additionally, they are frequently less expensive, and they may be useful for people who are new to just using dumbbells.

PART 3: HEALTH BENEFITS OF USING DUMBBELLS

Dumbbells may be used as part of a resistance workout regimen. Resistance conditioning can be done at least twice a week, according to the American Heart Association (AHA).

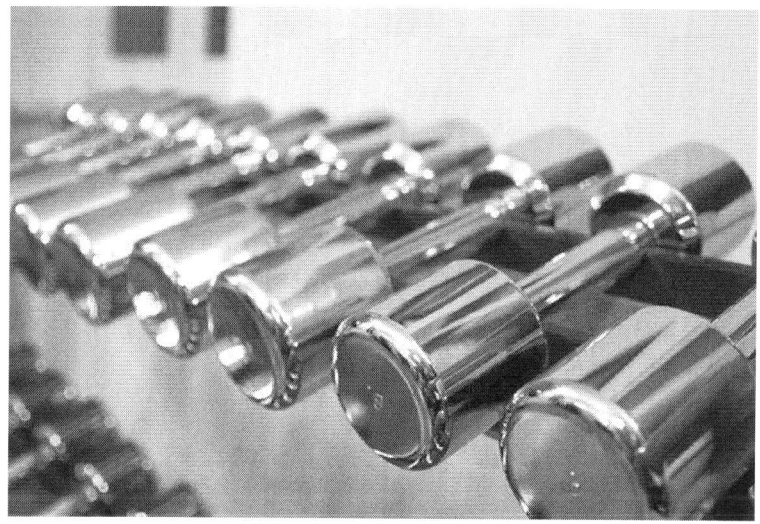

The followings are the health benefits of using Dumbbells for your workouts.

- It enhances resting metabolic rate.
- It burns calories faster.
- It enhances arms Muscles.
- Protecting against injuries.
- Increases strength also better for strength training.
- It is good for bodybuilding and fitness purposes.
- It helps to improve flexibility and mobility.
- It improves relaxation.
- It promotes coordination of muscles and stability.

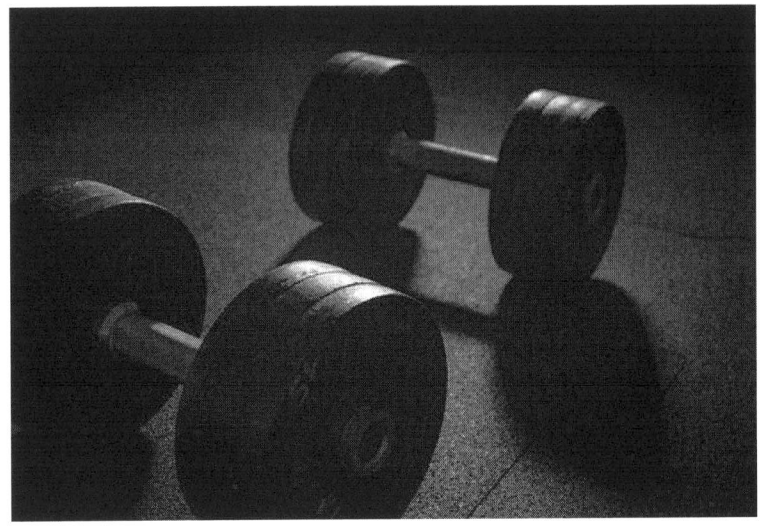

Other advantages are:

- It is portable.
- Easy to take along example traveling.
- It is flexible.
- More portable than Kettlebell.
- The adjustable dumbbells are suitable for beginners since they can be adjusted.
- Less expensive.

PART 4: HOW TO USE DUMBBELL FOR YOUR EXERCISES

Dumbbells can be utilized for a wide range of movements, including strength and cardio workouts. Dumbbells are one of the most flexible weights including they can be used to work the core, upper body, as well as the lower body all at the same time.

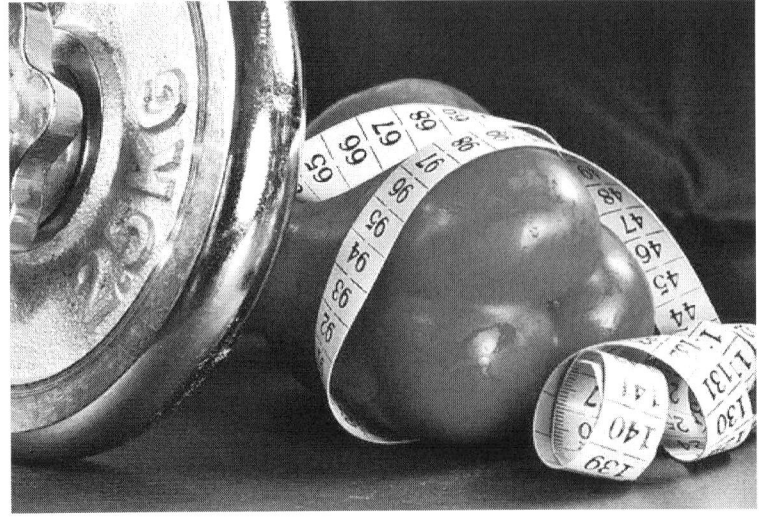

An individual should start with light weights but mostly practice the perfect technique for the workout they want to do. To avoid injuries, they should preserve good form and use proper technique.

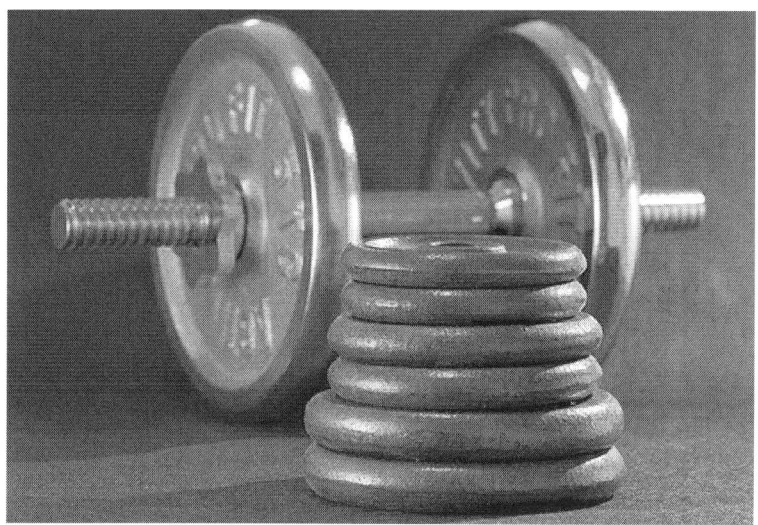

Once an individual is satisfied with the weight, they may raise it to render the movement more challenging. They can, though, stop if they fear the weight is out of balance or being too high.

PART 5: BEST DUMBBELL EXERCISES

The followings are the kind of workout performance that you can do with a dumbbell for your body fitness, Boost muscles, and effective body rehabilitation.

DUMBBELL BENCH PRESS:

- Lie straight on the bench.
- Ensure that your legs are bent and your feet are on the floor.
- Your dumbbell should be held tight with your hand strong.
- Raise it upward and downward.
- Repeat the process.
- 5-10 times.

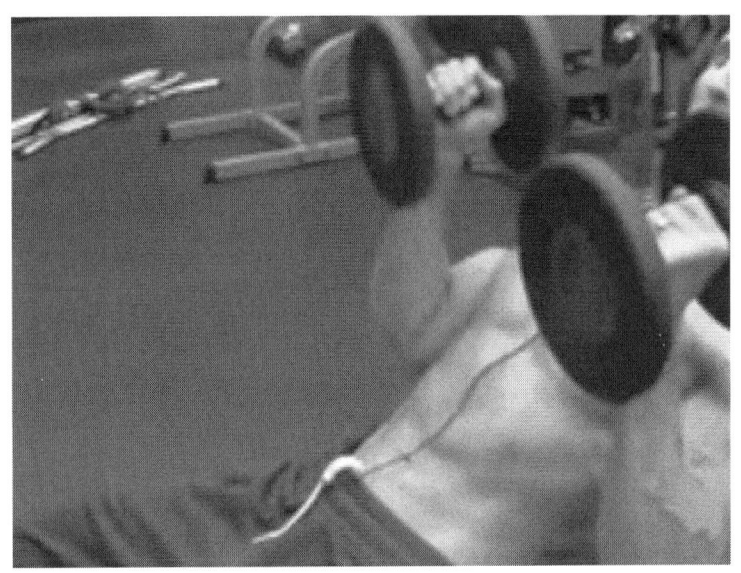

GOBLET SQUAT:

- First of all, stand straight.
- With your dumbbell held tight.
- Ensure that you hold the weight of the dumbbell with your two hands strong.
- Your legs should be a little bit wide.
- Squat downward and stand up to enable you to relocate to the original position.
- Repeat the same thing.

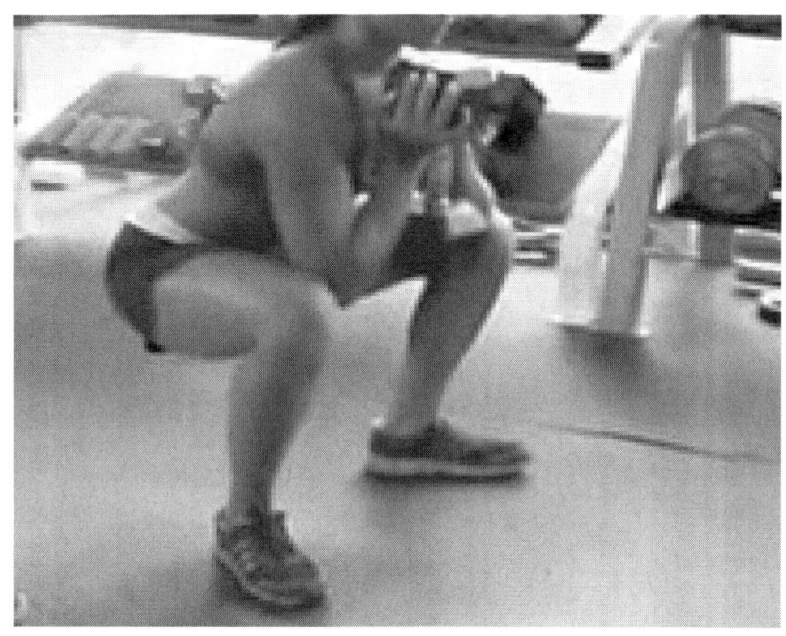

DUMBBELL CLEAN:

- Firstly stand straight.
- Your legs should be a little bit wide.
- And your dumbbell should be on the floor within your legs.
- Raise the dumbbell at your shoulder level.
- Back again to the original position.
- Repeat the same thing.

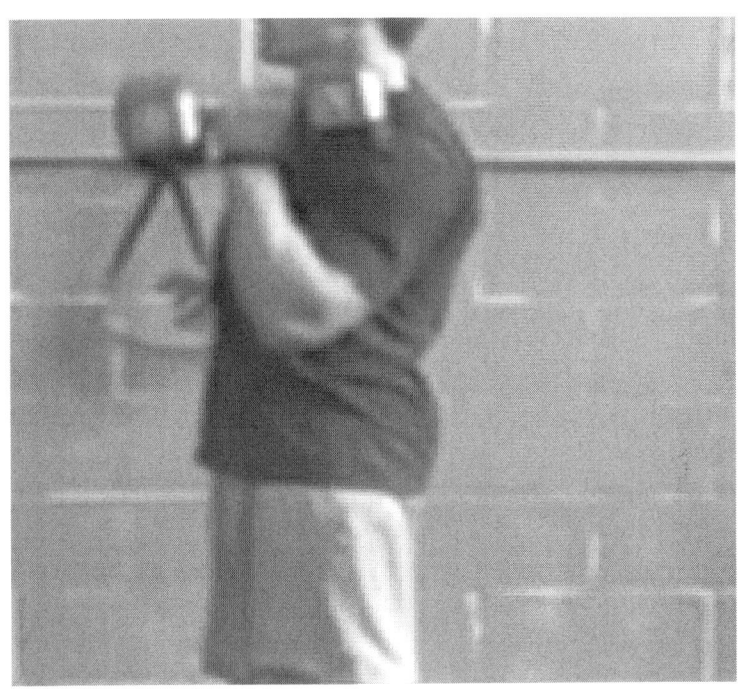

DUMBBELL BICEP CURL:

- Firstly, ensure you stand upright.
- Hold the dumbbell tight or strong with your palm.
- While you pull the dumbbell towards your chest.
- Release downward.
- Repeat the same.

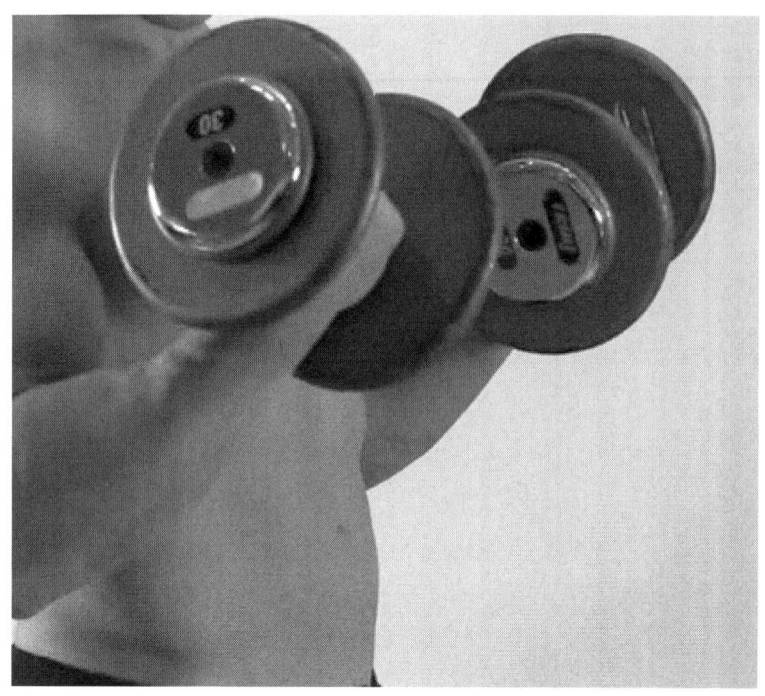

SHOULDER PRESS WITH DUMBBELL:

This is an excellent shoulder Exercises. If you like to strengthen your shoulders, the shoulder press mostly is the exercise for you. The Anterior Deltoid, Medial Deltoid, including the upper part of the Pectoralis Major is the specific muscles included.

- Firstly stand upright.
- With your dumbbell in your hand.

- Hold tight and lift it above your head level and your hands straight.
- Bring down at your shoulder level.

BEND OVER ROW:

- Stand on your feet.
- Bend 90 degrees downward with dumbbells on both hands.
- Pull the dumbbell upward towards your chest.
- Release your hand downward.
- Repeat the same.

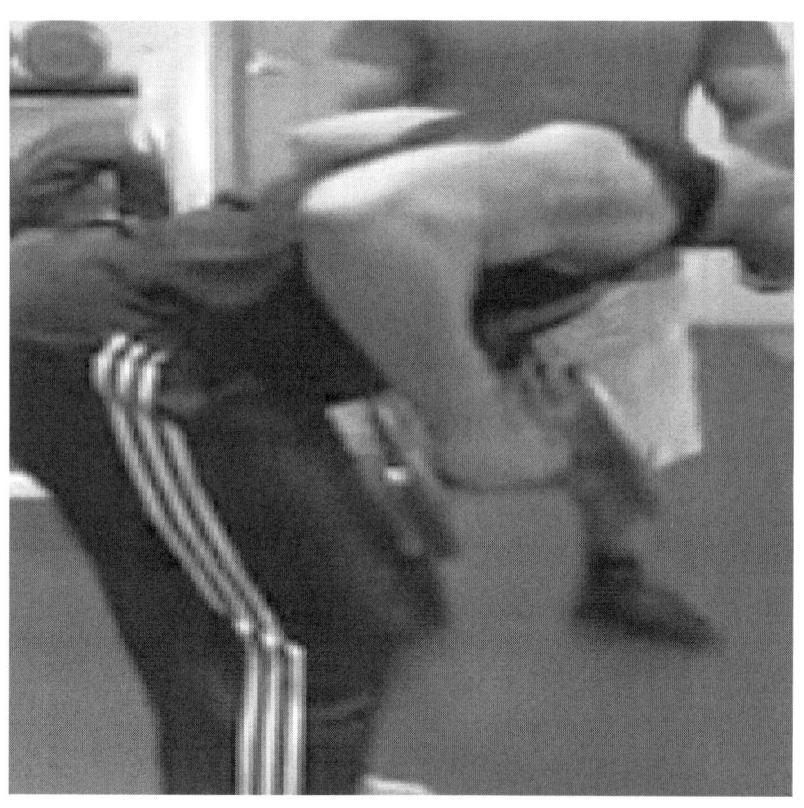

TWO-ARM DUMBBELL STIFF LEGGED DEADLIFT:

- Ensure that you hold tight two dumbbells.
- Let it be by your side and ensure that your knees are a little bit bent.
- Ensure that your lower side of the dumbbells to the top of your feet.

- to the degree that you can go by extending through your waist,
- Then little by little go back to the initial position.

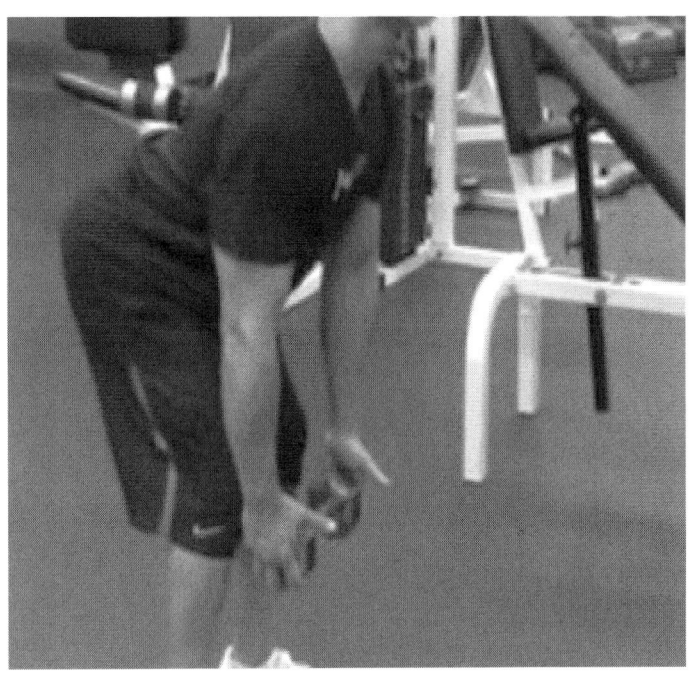

ONE-ARM SWING:

- Stand upright
- Ensure that your legs are a little bit open.
- Hold dumbbell one of your hand.
- While you swing it upward and downward.

- Repeat the same.

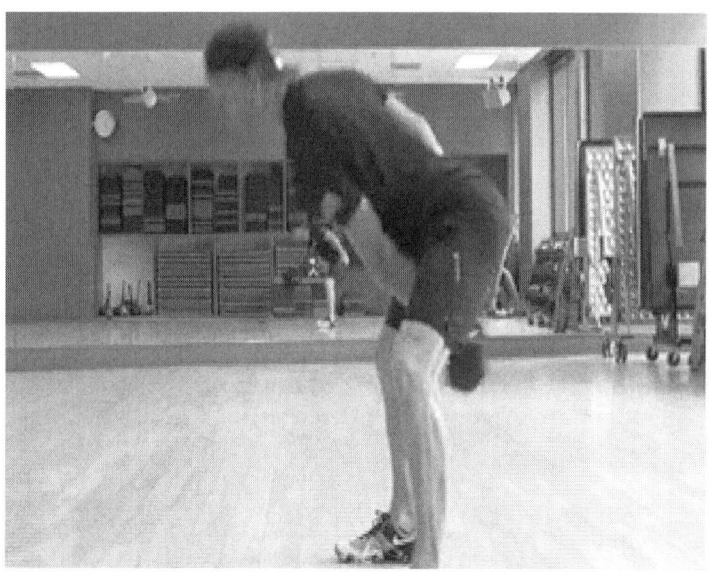

CROSSBODY SINGLE HAMMER CURL:

- Ensure that you curl each of the weights up against the opposing shoulder one at a time.
- .Adjust to the starting point under control and repeat on the other line.
- Note, if you like to build the arms race, you need to follow the divide as well as conquer strategy.

Concentrating on one arm at a time generates a large neuronal drive, causing the nervous system to attract more muscle fibers.

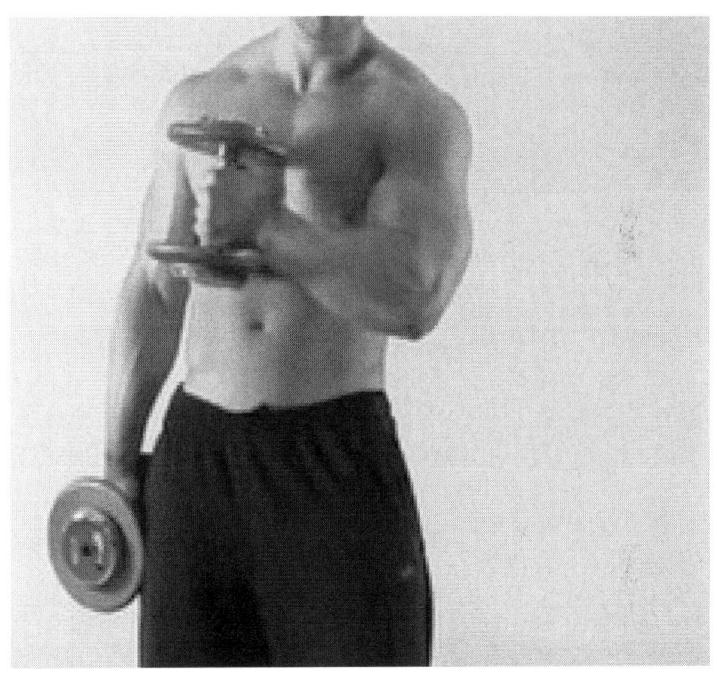

STEP-UPS WITH DUMBBELL:

Position your right foot mostly on the raised stage as well as pull yourself up by pushing up with your heel. Repeat with your left foot. Go down slowly with your left foot, focusing on flexing your right leg's hip as well as knee Rep on the other side.

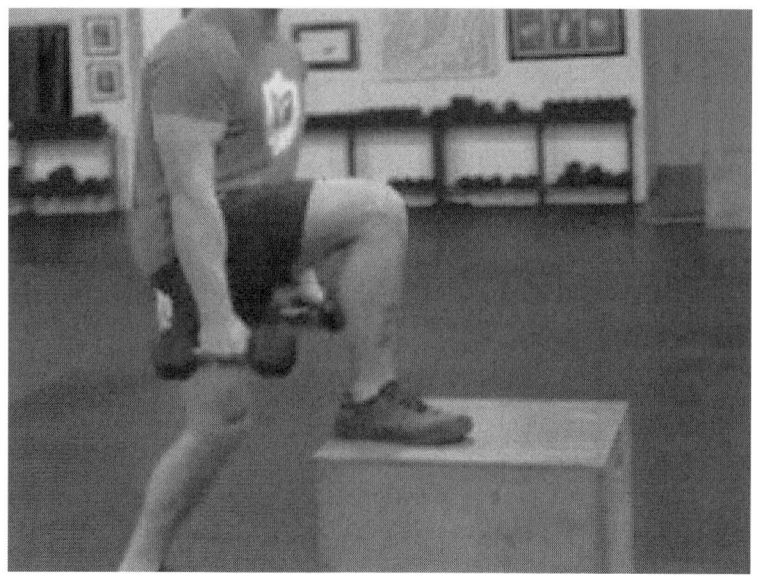

DUMBBELL SCAPTION:

Arc the weights up to your sides, arms upright, until you sense a heavy stretch over your shoulders. Back up to the starting spot.

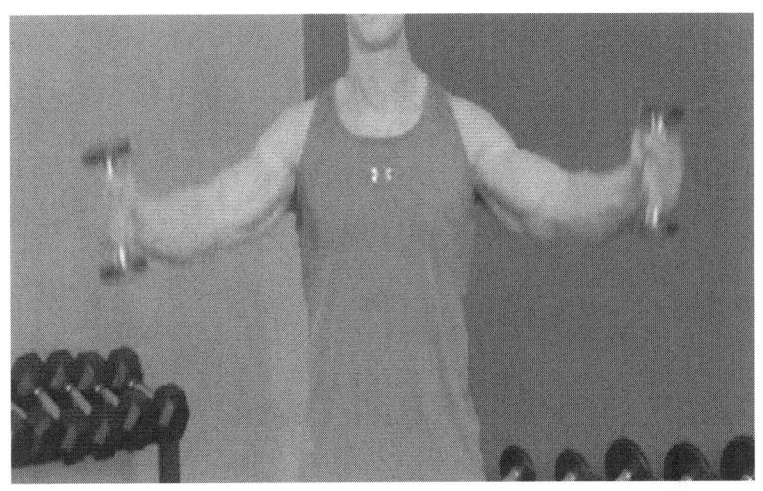

DUMBBELL LUNGE:

With your hands facing your body structure, place with dumbbells at your sides. Lunge forward or frontward at first with your right leg as hard as you can, lowering your trailing knee nearly to the concrete. Push your upper body back to the beginning point with the heel of your out-most right foot. Replace the opposite leg and repeat the process.

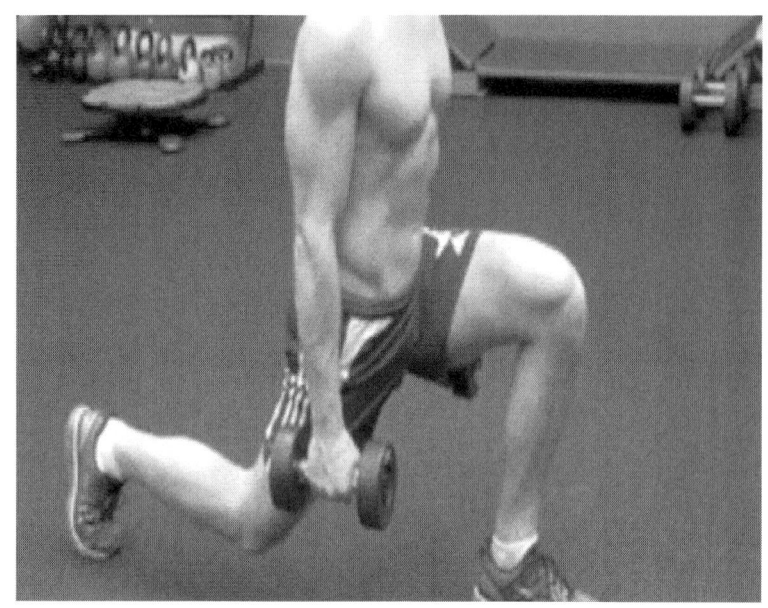

SINGLE DUMBBELL SHOULDER RAISE:

In both hands, hold the dumbbell at the edge as well as hang it across the thighs, shoulder-width apart. Lift the dumbbell straight or directly higher than your head while holding your arms out, then drop it and repeat.

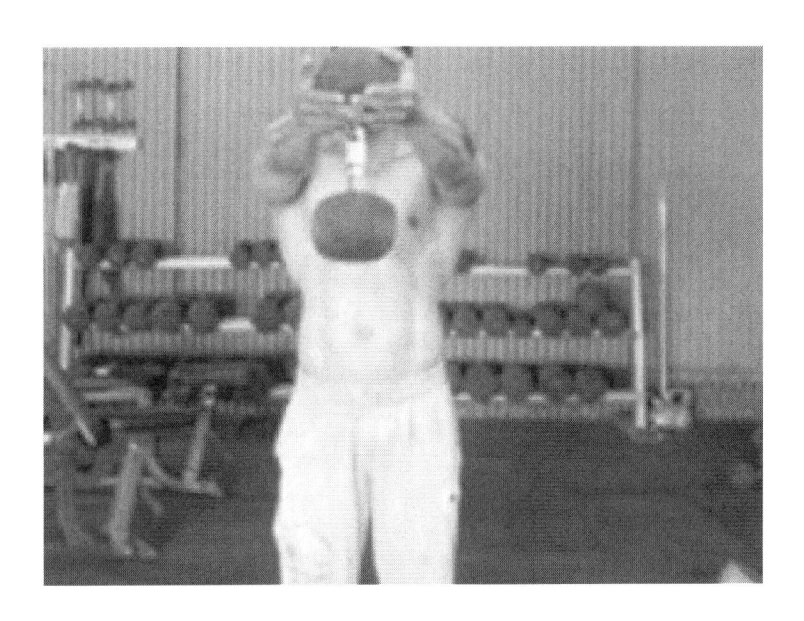

DUMBBELL CALF RAISES:

- Place a dumbbell in each hand as well as balance with your feet together.
- Around shoulder-width apart to do a calf raise with dumbbells.
- Allow your arms to dangle freely below your shoulders. When you rise to your knees, slowly return to your starting spot.
- Hold the back as well as knees straight while doing calf raises.

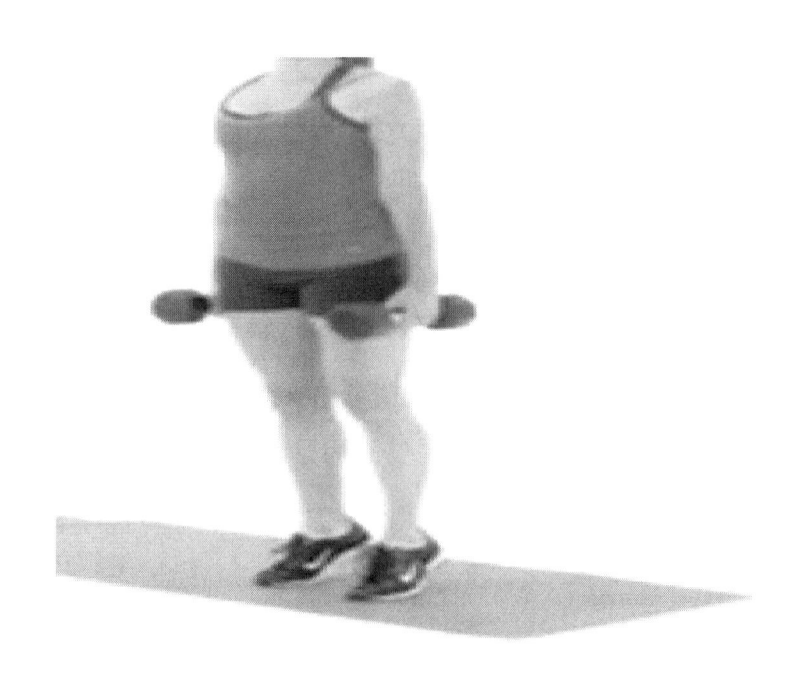

HOLLOW BODY SKULLCRUSHER:

Lie down on the ground with your back to the floor and your legs should be straight, with two dumbbells directly above your shoulders. Press your lower back touching the ground while tightening your abs. Lift your knees off the ground by an inch. Lift your shoulder blades over your head. Move your upper arms back slightly while you try to keep your arms straight. Lower the weights until they almost meet your shoulders, bending just at the elbows and holding the rest of the body secure in the starting spot. go again to the initial position, straightening just at the elbows.

TRICEP KICKBACK:

Starting with lighter weights and increasing the load as you progress is the best way to do this dumbbell workout. This is particularly true for the triceps kickback, a movement that targets the often-overlooked back of the arm. Using a spot close to the bent-over row, it's important to limit the movement to your lower arm alone. Throughout this movement, try to keep the shoulder as well as upper body.

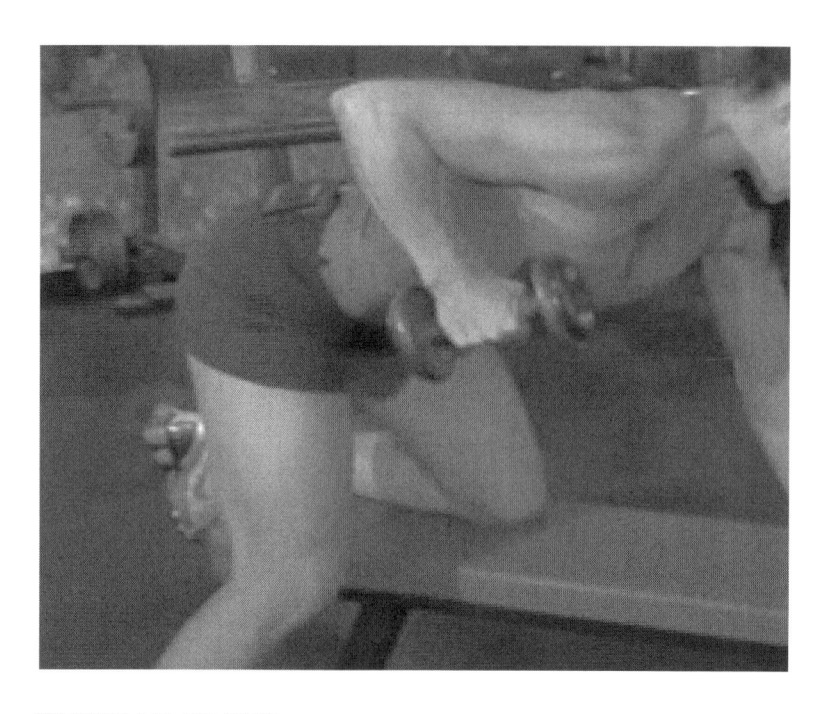

RUSSIAN TWIST:

- Lie straight on the floor.
- Raise your two legs and your back.
- Ensure that your legs and your back do not touch the ground.
- Hold the dumbbell with your two hands.
- While moving it to the right and the left side.
- Repeat the same.

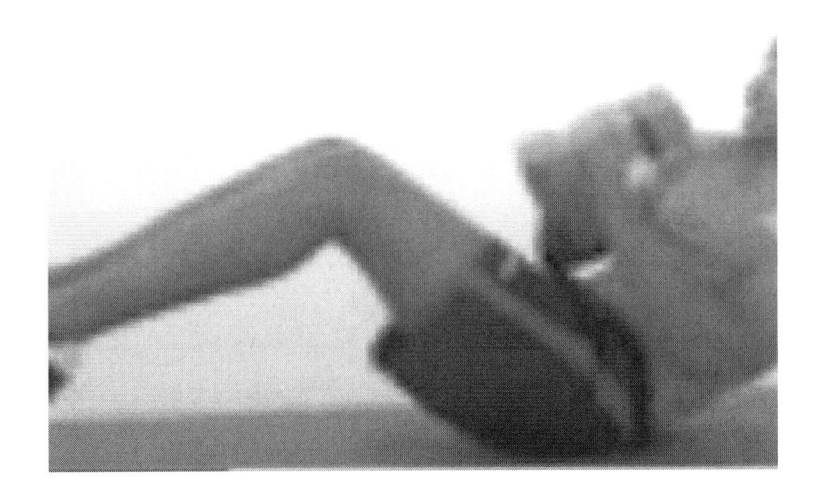

WEIGHT SIT UP/JACK KNIVE:

- Lie straight on the floor.
- Your feet need to be on the ground as well as your legs bent.
- Hold strong your dumbbell close or near to your chest with your two hands.
- Your back needs to be on the floor while you are performing push up.
- Repeat the same thing.

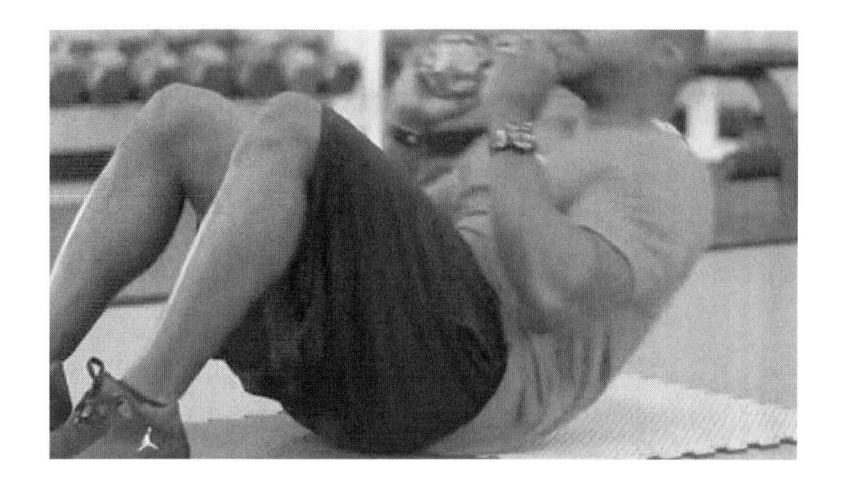

LATERAL RAISE DUMBBELL:

- Stand upright.
- Hold two dumbbells. One at your left as well as the other at your right hand.
- Raise your both hand sideward but not above your shoulder.
- Repeat the same.

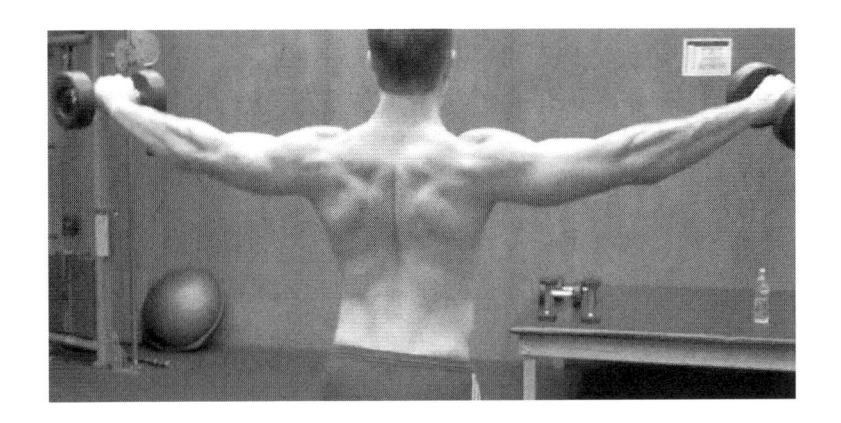

LYING DUMBBELL FLY:

- Lie straight on the bench with face facing up.
- With your back on the bench.
- The dumbbell should be on both hands.
- Raise the dumbbell upward above your body level.
- Release your arm back to the normal position.

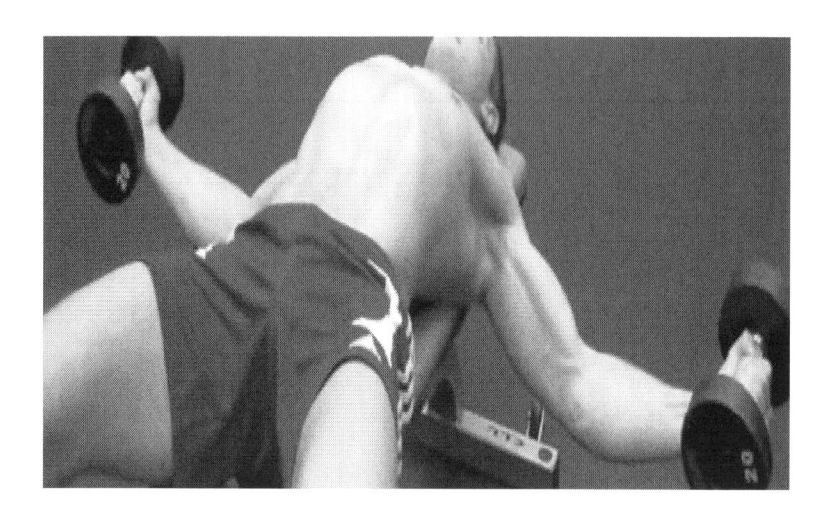

PRESS-UP WITH DUMBBELL:

- Lie straight on the floor.
- With your legs a little bit open and your face facing the toward the floor.
- Hold a tight dumbbell with your hand one at your left hand and the send at your right hand.
- Your kneels and your stomach should not touch the floor.
- While your hand should remain straight.
- Raised your left hand with the dumbbell while the other hand on the floor with a dumbbell.

- Do the same thing with your right hand.

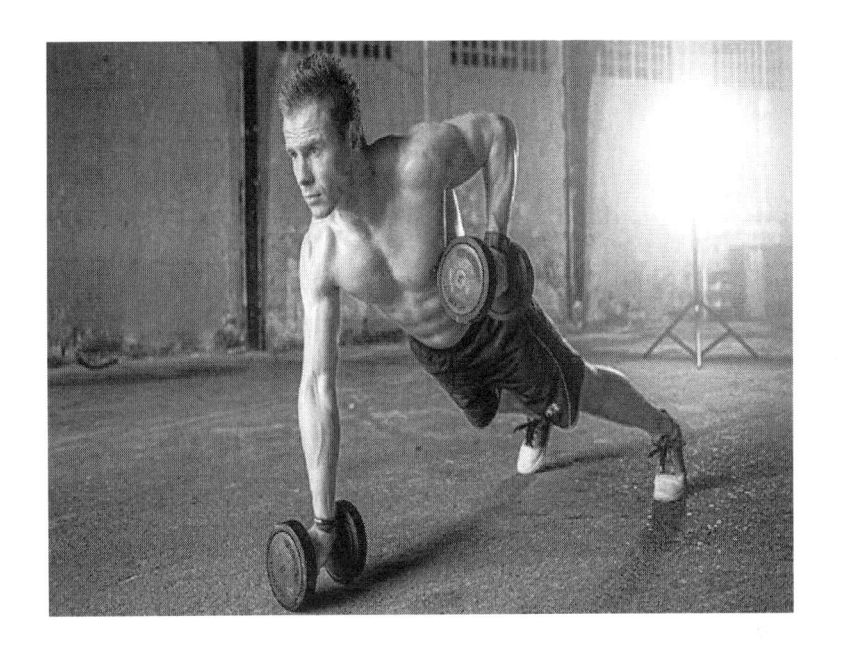

Printed in Dunstable, United Kingdom